The Complete Plant-Based Guide for Inspired Meals

Super Simple Plant-Based Cookbook for your family's Health

Ben Goleman

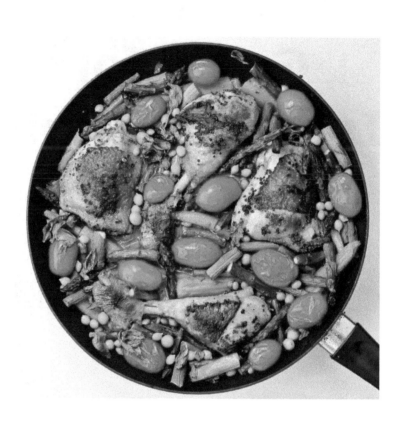

from various sources. Please consult a licensed professional before attempting any techniques outlined in this book.

By reading this document, the reader agrees that under no circumstances is the author responsible for any losses, direct or indirect, which are incurred as a result of the use of information contained within this document, including, but not limited to, — errors, omissions, or inaccuracies.

Table of Contents

Cashew Cream Cheese

Servings: 6

Cooking Time: 10 Minutes

Ingredients:

- 1 ½ cups cashews, soaked overnight and drained
- 1/3 cup water
- 1/4 teaspoon coarse sea salt
- 1/4 teaspoon dried dill weed
- 1/4 teaspoon garlic powder
- 2 tablespoons nutritional yeast
- 2 probiotic capsules

Directions:

1. Process the cashews and water in your blender until creamy and uniform.

2. Add in the salt, dill, garlic powder and nutritional yeast; continue to blend until everything is well incorporated.

3. Spoon the mixture into a sterilized glass jar. Add in the probiotic powder and combine with a wooden spoon (not metal!

4. Cover the jar with a clean kitchen towel and let it stand on the kitchen counter to ferment for 248 hours.

5.   Keep in your refrigerator for up to a week. Bon appétit!

Nutrition Info: Per Serving: Calories: 197; Fat: 14.4g;

Carbs: 11.4g; Protein: 7.4g

Avocado And Roasted Beet Salad

Servings: 2

Cooking Time: 40 Minutes

Ingredients:

- 2 beets, thinly sliced and peeled
- 1 teaspoon of olive oil
- A pinch of sea salt
- 1 avocado
- 2 cups of mixed greens
- 4 tablespoons of creamy Balsamic Dressing
- 2 tablespoons of chopped almonds

Directions:

1. Prepare the oven by preheating it to 450 degrees F.
2. In a large bowl, combine the oil, beets and salt, massage with your hands.
3. Arrange the beets in a single layer on a baking dish and bake them for minutes.
4. Slice the avocado in half and remove the seed.
5. Scoop out the avocado flesh in one piece and slice it into crescents.

6. Once the beets are cooked, remove them from the oven and arrange the slices onto plates.

7. Top the beets with a slice of avocado, a handful of salad and drizzle the dressing over the top, coat with some chopped almonds and serve.

Vegan Bake Pasta with Bolognese Sauce and Cashew Cream

Servings: 8

Cooking Time: 20 Minutes

Ingredients:

- For the Pasta:
- 1 packet penne pasta
- For the Bolognese Sauce:
- 1 tablespoon soy sauce
- 1 small can lentils
- 1 tablespoon brown sugar
- ½ cup tomato paste
- 1 teaspoon garlic, crushed
- 1 tablespoon olive oil
- 2 tomatoes, chopped
- 1 onion, chopped
- 2 cups mushrooms, sliced
- Salt, to taste
- Pepper, to taste
- For the Cashew Cream:
- 1 cup raw cashews
- ½ lemon, squeezed
- ½ teaspoon salt

- ½ cup water

- For the White Sauce:

- 1 teaspoon black pepper

- 1 teaspoon Dijon mustard

- ¼ cup nutritional yeast

- Sea salt, as required

- 2 cups coconut milk

- 3 tablespoons vegan butter

- 2 tablespoons all-purpose flour

- 1/3 cup vegetable broth

Directions:

1. Take a pot and boil water, add pasta to it, boil for 3 minutes and set aside.

2. Fry onion and garlic, mushroom in olive oil and add soy sauce to it.

3. Add in sugar tomato paste, lentils, and canned tomato to it and let it simmer, Bolognese sauce is prepared.

4. Season it with salt and black pepper.

5. Add the lemon juice, cashews, water and salt to the blender, blend for 2 minutes.

6. Add this to the sauce you have prepared and stir pasta in it.

7. Melt the vegan butter in a saucepan, add in the flour and stir.

8. Add vegetable stock and coconut milk to it and whisk well.

9. Stir continuously and let it boil for about 5 minutes, then remove from heat.

10. Add Dijon mustard, nutritional yeast, black pepper, and sea salt.

11. Preheat the oven to 430 degrees F.

12. Prepare rectangular oven-safe dish by placing pasta and Bolognese sauce to it.

13. Pour the white sauce on it and bake for a time period of 20-25 minutes.

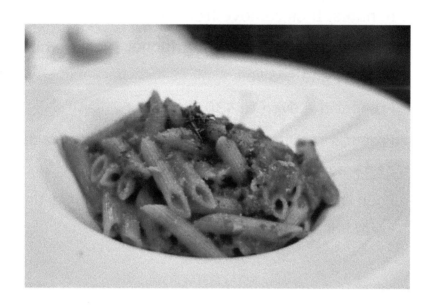

Maple Green Cabbage Hash

Servings: 4

Cooking Time: 25 Minutes

Ingredients:

- 3 tbsp olive oil
- 2 shallots, thinly sliced
- 1 ½ lb green cabbage, shredded
- 3 tbsp apple cider vinegar
- 1 tbsp pure maple syrup
- ½ tsp sriracha sauce

Directions:

1. Heat the oil in a skillet over medium heat. Place in shallots and cabbage and cook for minutes until tender. Pour in vinegar and scrape any bits from the bottom. Mix in maple syrup and sriracha sauce. Cook for 3-5 minutes, until the liquid absorbs. Sprinkle with salt and pepper.

Serve right away.

Zesty Rice Bowls with Tempeh

Servings: 4

Cooking Time: 50 Minutes

Ingredients:

- 2 tbsp olive oil
- 1 ½ cups crumbled tempeh
- 1 tsp Creole seasoning
- 2 red bell peppers, sliced
- 1 cup brown rice
- 2 cups vegetable broth
- Salt to taste
- 1 lemon, zested and juiced
- 1 (8 oz) can black beans, drained
- 2 chives, chopped
- 2 tbsp freshly chopped parsley

Directions:

1. Heat the olive oil in a medium pot and cook in the tempeh until golden brown, 5 minutes. Season with the Creole seasoning and stir in the bell peppers. Cook until the peppers slightly soften, 3 minutes. Stir in the brown rice, vegetable broth, salt, and lemon zest. Cover and cook until the rice is tender and all the liquid is absorbed,

to 25 minutes. Mix in the lemon juice, beans, and chives. Allow warming for 3 to 5 minutes and dish the food. Garnish with the parsley and serve warm.

Butternut Squash Steak

Servings: 4

Cooking Time: 50 Minutes

Ingredients:

- 2 tbsp. coconut yogurt
- ½ t. sweet paprika
- 1 ¼ c. low-sodium vegetable broth
- 1 sprig thyme
- 1 finely chopped garlic clove
- 1 big thinly sliced shallot
- 1 tbsp. margarine
- 2 tbsp. olive oil, extra virgin
- Salt and pepper to liking

Directions:

1. Bring the oven to 375 heat setting.
2. Cut the squash, lengthwise, into 4 steaks.
3. Carefully core one side of each squash with a paring knife in a crosshatch pattern.
4. Using a brush, coat with olive oil each side of the steak then season generously with salt and pepper.

5.   In an oven-safe, non-stick skillet, bring 2 tablespoons of olive oil to a warm temperature.

6.   Place the steaks on the skillet with the cored side down and cook at medium temperature until browned, approximately 5 minutes.

7.   Flip and repeat on the other side for about 3 minutes.

8.   Place the skillet into the oven to roast the squash for 7 minutes.

9.   Take out from the oven, placing on a plate and covering with aluminum foil to keep warm.

10.   Using the previously used skillet, add thyme, garlic, and shallot, cooking at medium heat. Stir frequently for about 2 minutes.

11.   Add brandy and cook for an additional minute.

12.   Next, add paprika and whisk the mixture together for 3 minutes.

13.   Add in the yogurt seasoning with salt and pepper.

14.   Plate the steaks and spoon the sauce over the top.

15.   Garnish with parsley and enjoy!

Nutrition Info: Calories: 300 Carbohydrates: 46 g Proteins: 5.3 g Fats: 10.6g

Garlic And Lemon Mushroom Salad

Servings: 2

Cooking Time: 10 Minutes

Ingredients:

- 8 ounces mushrooms
- 1/2 teaspoon garlic powder
- 1 tablespoon chopped parsley
- 1 teaspoon soy sauce
- ½ teaspoon salt
- 1/3 teaspoon ground black pepper
- 2 tablespoons olive oil
- 2 wedges of lemon for serving

Directions:

1. Switch on the air fryer, insert the fryer basket, then shut it with the lid, set the frying temperature 380 degrees F, and let it preheat for 5 minutes.

2. Meanwhile, cut mushrooms in quarters, then place them in a bowl, add remaining ingredients, except for lemon wedges and toss until coated.

3. Open the preheated fryer, place mushrooms in it, close the lid and cook for 10 minutes until golden brown and cooked, shaking halfway.

4.   When done, the air fryer will beep, open the lid, and transfer mushrooms to the salad bowls.

5.   Let mushroom cool for 10 minutes and then serve straight away.

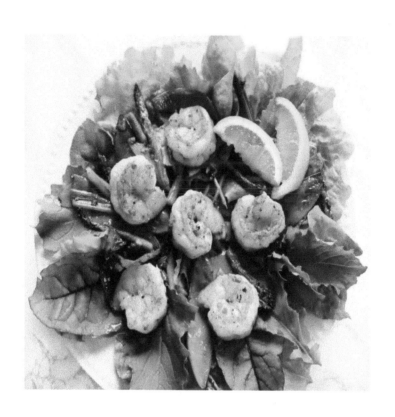

Vegan Mushroom Pizza

Servings: 4

Cooking Time: 35 Minutes

Ingredients:

- 2 tsp plant butter
- 1 cup chopped button mushrooms
- ½ cup sliced mixed bell peppers
- Salt and black pepper to taste
- 1 pizza crust
- 1 cup tomato sauce
- 1 cup plant-based Parmesan cheese
- 5-6 basil leaves

Directions:

1. Melt plant butter in a skillet and sauté mushrooms and bell peppers for minutes until soften. Season with salt and black pepper. Put the pizza crust on a pizza pan, spread the tomato sauce all over and scatter vegetables evenly on top. Sprinkle with plant-based Parmesan cheese. Bake for 20 minutes until the cheese has melted.

Garnish with basil, slice and serve.

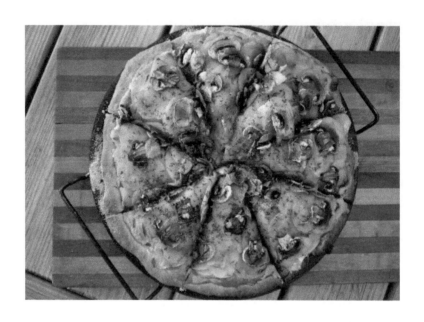

Harissa Bulgur Bowl

Servings: 4

Cooking Time: 25 Minutes

Ingredients:

- 1 cup bulgur wheat
- 1 ½ cups vegetable broth
- 2 cups sweet corn kernels, thawed
- 1 cup canned kidney beans, drained
- 1 red onion, thinly sliced
- 1 garlic clove, minced
- Sea salt and ground black pepper, to taste
- 1/4 cup harissa paste
- 1 tablespoon lemon juice
- 1 tablespoon white vinegar
- 1/4 cup extra-virgin olive oil
- 1/4 cup fresh parsley leaves, roughly chopped

Directions:

1. In a deep saucepan, bring the bulgur wheat and vegetable broth to a simmer; let it cook, covered, for to 13 minutes.

2. Let it stand for 5 to 10 minutes and fluff your bulgur with a fork.

3.   Add the remaining ingredients to the cooked bulgur wheat; serve warm or at room temperature. Bon appétit!

Nutrition Info: Per Serving: Calories: 353; Fat: 15.5g;

Carbs: 48.5g; Protein: 8.4g

Crunchy Asparagus Spears

Servings: 4

Cooking Time: 25 Minutes

Ingredients:

- 1 bunch asparagus spears (about 12 spears)
- ¼ cup nutritional yeast
- 2 tablespoons hemp seeds
- 1 teaspoon garlic powder
- ¼ teaspoon paprika (or more if you like paprika)
- ⅛ teaspoon ground pepper
- ¼ cup whole-wheat breadcrumbs
- Juice of ½ lemon

Directions:

1. Preheat the oven to 350 degrees, Fahrenheit. Line a baking sheet with parchment paper.

2. Wash the asparagus, snapping off the white part at the bottom. Save it for making vegetable stock.

3. Mix together the nutritional yeast, hemp seed, garlic powder, paprika, pepper and breadcrumbs.

4. Place asparagus spears on the baking sheets giving them a little room in between and sprinkle with the mixture in the bowl.

5. Bake for up to 2minutes, until crispy.

6. Serve with lemon juice if desired.

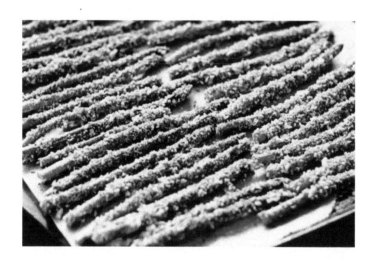

Grilled Tofu with Chimichurri Sauce

Servings: 4

Cooking Time: 12 Minutes

Ingredients:

- 2 tablespoons plus 1 teaspoon olive oil
- 1 teaspoon dried oregano
- 1 cup parsley leaves
- ½ cup cilantro leaves
- 2 Fresno peppers, seeded and chopped
- 2 tablespoons white wine vinegar
- 2 tablespoons water
- 1 tablespoon fresh lime juice
- Salt and black pepper
- 1 cup couscous, cooked
- 1 teaspoon lime zest
- ¼ cup toasted pumpkin seeds
- 1 cup fresh spinach, chopped
- 1 (15.5 ounce) can kidney beans, rinsed and drained
- 1 (14 to 16 ounce) block tofu, diced
- 2 summer squashes, diced
- 3 spring onions, quartered

Directions:

1. In a saucepan, heat 2 tablespoons oil and add oregano over medium heat.

2. After 30 seconds add parsley, chili pepper, cilantro, lime juice, tablespoons water, vinegar, salt and black pepper.

3. Mix well then blend in a blender.

4. Add the remining oil, pumpkin seeds, beans and spinach and cook for 3 minutes.

5. Stir in couscous and adjust seasoning with salt and black pepper.

6. Prepare and set up a grill on medium heat.

7. Thread the tofu, squash, and onions on the skewer in an alternating pattern.

8. Grill these skewers for 4 minutes per side while basting with the green sauce.

9. Serve the skewers on top of the couscous with green sauce.

10. Enjoy.

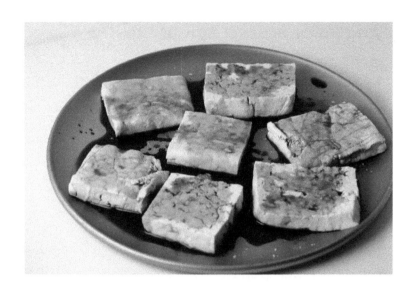

Sweet And Spicy Brussel Sprout Stir-fry

Servings: 4

Cooking Time: 15 Minutes

Ingredients:

- 4 oz plant butter + more to taste
- 4 shallots, chopped
- 1 tbsp apple cider vinegar
- Salt and black pepper to taste
- 1 lb Brussels sprouts
- Hot chili sauce

Directions:

1. Put the plant butter in a saucepan and melt over medium heat. Pour in the shallots and sauté for 2 minutes, to caramelize and slightly soften.

2. Add the apple cider vinegar, salt, and black pepper. Stir and reduce the heat to cook the shallots further with continuous stirring, about 5 minutes. Transfer to a plate after.

3. Trim the Brussel sprouts and cut in halves. Leave the small ones as wholes. Pour the Brussel sprouts into the saucepan and stir-fry with more plant butter until softened but al dente. Season with salt and black

pepper, stir in the onions and hot chili sauce, and heat for a few seconds. Serve immediately.

Tasty Salad with Lentil & Red Onion and A Dash of Roasted Cumin

Servings: 3

Cooking Time: 35 Minutes

Ingredients:

- 2 cans of green lentils
- 70 g of watercress
- 20 g of coriander
- 4 carrots
- 2 teaspoons of fennel seeds •   2 red onions
- 2 teaspoons of cumin seeds
- 50 g of pine nuts
- Olive oil
- Cashew cheese:
- 1 freshly juiced lemon
- Salt
- 150 g of cashew nuts
- Pepper
- 5 tablespoons of water

Directions:

1.   Preheat the oven to 0o C. Peel the carrots and slice them diagonally. Roughly chop the onions.

2.   Put the carrots and onion on a baking tray and sprinkle with cumin and fennel seeds. Do not forget a good dose of olive oil on the top. Top with salt and pepper. Roast everything in the oven for half an hour.

3.   Heat a pan and fry the pine nuts without oil. Once they start to brown, take them off the stove and allow them to cool.

4.   Put all of the ingredients for the cashew cheese in a blender and create a smooth puree.

5.   Once the veggies are cooked, rinse the lentils and add them to a warm pan. They should be slightly warm. Add the carrots and onion with the seeds. Scoop some oil from the baking tray and include it in this mixture as well. 6. Chop the coriander roughly and add it to the lentil mixture. Season with salt and pepper to taste.

7.   Remove the pan from the heat and add the watercress. Plate the salad with a good sprinkle of pine nuts on top.

8.   Top the salad with some good cashew cheese and enjoy this fresh, amazing salad, which is the best remedy for an empty stomach.

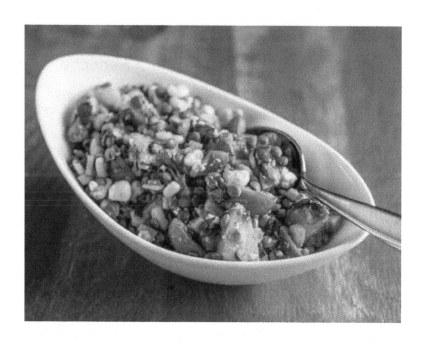

Spaghetti Squash In Tahini Sauce

Servings: 4

Cooking Time: 50 Minutes

Ingredients:

- 1 (3-pound) spaghetti squash, halved lengthwise
- 1 tbsp rice vinegar
- 1 tbsp tahini
- Salt and black pepper to taste

Directions:

1. Preheat oven to 390 F. Line with parchment paper a baking sheet. Slice the squash half lengthwise and arrange on the baking sheet skin-side up. Bake for 3540 minutes. Let cool before scraping the flesh to make "noodles". Place the spaghetti in a bowl. In another bowl whisk tbsp hot water, vinegar, tahini, salt, and pepper. Add into the spaghetti bowl and toss to coat. Serve.

Pungent Mushroom Barley Risotto

Servings: 4

Cooking Time: 3 Hours And 9 Minutes

Ingredients:

- 1 1/2 cups of hulled barley, rinsed and soaked overnight
- 8 ounces of carrots, peeled and chopped • 1 pound of mushrooms, sliced
- 1 large white onion, peeled and chopped
- 3/4 teaspoon of salt
- 1/2 teaspoon of ground black pepper
- 4 sprigs thyme
- 1/4 cup of chopped parsley
- 2/3 cup of grated vegan Parmesan cheese
- 1 tablespoon of apple cider vinegar
- 2 tablespoons of olive oil
- 1 1/2 cups of vegetable broth

Directions:

1. Place a large non-stick skillet pan over a mediumhigh heat, add the oil and let it heat until it gets hot.

2. Add the onion along with 1/4 teaspoon of each the salt and black pepper.

3. Cook it for 5 minutes or until it turns golden brown.

4. Then add the mushrooms and continue cooking for 2 minutes.

5. Add the barley, thyme and cook for another 2 minutes.

6. Transfer this mixture to a quarts slow cooker and add the carrots, 1/4 teaspoon of salt, and the vegetable broth.

7. Stir properly and cover it with the lid.

8. Plug in the slow cooker, let it cook for 3 hours at the high heat setting or until the grains absorb all the cooking liquid and the vegetables get soft.

9. Remove the thyme sprigs, pour in the remaining ingredients except for parsley and stir properly.

10. Pour in the warm water and stir properly until the risotto reaches your desired state.

11. Add the seasoning, then garnish it with parsley and serve.

Nutrition Info: Calories:321 Cal, Carbohydrates:48g, Protein:12g, Fats:10g, Fiber:11g.

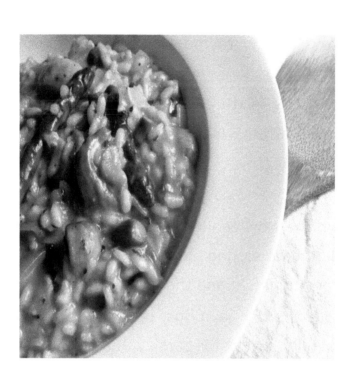

Sautéed Sesame Spinach

Servings: 4

Cooking Time: 3 Minutes

Ingredients:

- 1 tablespoon toasted sesame oil
- ½ tablespoon soy sauce
- ½ teaspoon toasted sesame seeds, crushed
- ½ teaspoon rice vinegar
- ½ teaspoon golden caster sugar
- 1 garlic clove, grated
- 8 ounces spinach, stem ends trimmed

Directions:

1. Sauté spinach in a pan until it is wilted.
2. Whisk the sesame oil, garlic, sugar, vinegar, sesame seeds, soy sauce and black pepper together in a bowl.
3. Stir in spinach and mix well.
4. Cover and refrigerate for 1 hour.
5. Serve.

Asparagus With Creamy Puree

Servings: 4

Cooking Time: 15 Minutes

Ingredients:

- 4 tbsp flax seed powder
- 2 oz plant butter, melted
- 3 oz cashew cream cheese
- ½ cup coconut cream
- Powdered chili pepper to taste
- 1 tbsp olive oil
- ½ lb asparagus, hard stalks removed
- 3 oz plant butter
- Juice of ½ a lemon

Directions:

1. In a safe microwave bowl, mix the flax seed powder with ½ cup water and set aside to thicken for 5 minutes. Warm the flax egg in the microwave for 2 minutes, then, pour into a blender. Add in plant butter, cashew cream cheese, coconut cream, salt, and chili pepper. Puree until smooth.

2. Heat olive oil in a saucepan and roast the asparagus until lightly charred. Season with salt and

black pepper and set aside. Melt plant butter in a frying pan until nutty and golden brown. Stir in lemon juice and pour the mixture into a sauce cup. Spoon the creamy blend into the center of four serving plates and use the back of the spoon to spread out lightly. Top with the asparagus and drizzle the lemon butter on top. Serve immediately.

Breaded Tofu Steaks

Servings: 4

Cooking Time: 12 Minutes

Ingredients:

- 3 cups (750 grams) tofu, extra-firm, pressed
- 4 tablespoons tomato paste
- 2 ½ tablespoons minced garlic
- 1 cup (236 grams) panko breadcrumbs and more as needed
- ½ teaspoon ground black pepper
- 2 tablespoon maple syrup
- 2 tablespoon Dijon mustard
- 2 tablespoon soy sauce
- 4 tablespoons olive oil
- 2 tablespoon water
- BBQ sauce for serving

Directions:

1. Prepare the tofu steaks: pat dry tofu and then cut them into four slices.
2. Prepare the sauce: take a medium bowl, add garlic, black pepper, maple syrup, mustard,

tomato paste, soy sauce, and water; stir until combined.

3.   Take a shallow dish and place bread crumbs on it.

4.   Working on one tofu steak at a time, first coat it with prepared sauce, then dredge it with bread crumbs until evenly coated and place it on a plate.

5.   Repeat with the remaining tofu slices.

6.   Take a frying pan, place it over medium heat, pour oil in it and when hot, place a tofu steak inside and cook for 4 to minutes per side until golden brown and cooked. 7. Transfer tofu steak to a plate and repeat with the remaining tofu steaks.

8.   Serve tofu steaks with the BBQ sauce.

Nutrition Info: 419.4 Cal; 23.9 g Fat; 3.9 g Saturated Fat; 33.3 g Carbs; 4.3 g Fiber; 22.8 g Protein; 3 g Sugar;

Chickpea & Bean Patties

Servings: 4

Cooking Time: 30 Minutes

Ingredients:

- 1 (15 oz) can chickpea, drained
- 1 (15 oz) can pinto beans, drained
- 1 (15 oz) can red kidney beans
- 2 tbsp whole-wheat flour
- ¼ cup dried mixed herbs
- ¼ tsp hot sauce
- ½ tsp garlic powder
- Salt and black pepper to taste
- 4 slices cashew cheese
- 4 whole-grain hamburger buns, split
- 4 small lettuce leaves for topping

Directions:

1.   In a medium bowl, mash the chickpea, pinto beans, kidney beans and mix in the flour, mixed herbs, hot sauce, garlic powder, salt, and black pepper. Mold 4 patties out of the mixture and set aside.

2.   Heat a grill pan to medium heat and grease with cooking spray. Cook the bean patties on both sides until

light brown and cooked through, 10 minutes. Lay a cashew cheese slice on each and allow slight melting, minutes. Remove the patties between the burger buns and top with the lettuce and serve.

Oven Baked Sesame Fries

Servings: 4

Cooking Time: 30 Minutes

Ingredients:

- 1 pound Yukon Gold potatoes, skins on and cut into wedges
- 2 tablespoons sesame seeds
- 1 tablespoon potato starch
- 1 tablespoon sesame oil
- Salt to taste
- Black pepper to taste

Directions:

1. Preheat the oven to 425 degrees, Fahrenheit and cover a baking sheet or two with parchment paper.
2. Cut the potatoes and place in a large bowl.
3. Add the sesame seeds, potato starch, sesame oil, salt and pepper.
4. Toss with your hands and make sure all the wedges are coated. Add more sesame seeds or oil if needed.

5.   Spread the potato wedges on the baking sheets with some room between each wedge.

6.   Bake for 15 minutes, flip the wedges over and then return them to the oven for 10 to 15 more minutes, until they look golden and crispy.

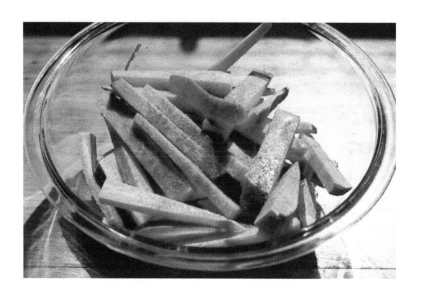

Aromatic Rice Pudding with Dried Figs

Servings: 4

Cooking Time: 45 Minutes

Ingredients:

- 2 cups water
- 1 cup medium-grain white rice
- 3 ½ cups coconut milk
- 1/2 cup coconut sugar
- 1 cinnamon stick
- 1 vanilla bean
- 1/2 cup dried figs, chopped
- 4 tablespoons coconut, shredded

Directions:

1.   In a saucepan, bring the water to a boil over medium-high heat. Immediately turn the heat to a simmer, add in the rice and let it cook for about 20 minutes.

2.   Add in the milk, sugar and spices and continue to cook for minutes more, stirring constantly to prevent the rice from sticking to the pan.

3.   Top with dried figs and coconut; serve your pudding warm or at room temperature. Bon appétit!

Nutrition Info: Per Serving: Calories: 407; Fat: 7.5g;
Carbs: 74.3g; Protein: 10.7g

Buckwheat Pilaf with Pine Nuts

Servings: 4

Cooking Time: 25 Minutes

Ingredients:

*   1 cup buckwheat groats
*   2 cups vegetable stock
*   ¼ cup pine nuts
*   2 tbsp olive oil
*   ½ onion, chopped
*   ⅓ cup chopped fresh parsley

Directions:

1.   Put the groats and vegetable stock in a pot. Bring to a boil, then lower the heat and simmer for minutes. Heat a skillet over medium heat. Place in the pine nuts and toast for 2-3 minutes, shaking often. Heat the oil in the same skillet and sauté the onion for 3 minutes until translucent.

2.   Once the groats are ready, fluff them using a fork. Mix in pine nuts, onion and parsley. Sprinkle with salt and pepper. Serve immediately.

Overnight Oatmeal with Prunes

Servings: 2

Cooking Time: 5 Minutes

Ingredients:

- 1 cup hemp milk
- 1 tablespoon flax seed, ground
- 2/3 cup rolled oats
- 2 ounces prunes, sliced
- 2 tablespoons agave syrup
- A pinch of salt
- 1/2 teaspoon ground cinnamon

Directions:

1. Divide the ingredients, except for the prunes, between two mason jars.
2. Cover and shake to combine well. Let them sit overnight in your refrigerator.
3. Garnish with sliced prunes just before serving.

Enjoy!

Nutrition Info: Per Serving: Calories: 398; Fat: 9.9g; Carbs: 66.2g; Protein: 13.7g

Chickpea Garden Vegetable Medley

Servings: 4

Cooking Time: 30 Minutes

Ingredients:

- 2 tablespoons olive oil
- 1 onion, finely chopped
- 1 bell pepper, chopped
- 1 fennel bulb, chopped
- 3 cloves garlic, minced
- 2 ripe tomatoes, pureed
- 2 tablespoons fresh parsley, roughly chopped
- 2 tablespoons fresh basil, roughly chopped
- 2 tablespoons fresh coriander, roughly chopped
- 2 cups vegetable broth
- 14 ounces canned chickpeas, drained
- Kosher salt and ground black pepper, to taste
- 1/2 teaspoon cayenne pepper
- 1 teaspoon paprika
- 1 avocado, peeled and sliced

Directions:

1.   In a heavy-bottomed pot, heat the olive oil over medium heat. Once hot, sauté the onion, bell pepper and fennel bulb for about 4 minutes.

2.   Sauté the garlic for about 1 minute or until aromatic.

3.   Add in the tomatoes, fresh herbs, broth, chickpeas, salt, black pepper, cayenne pepper and paprika. Let it simmer, stirring occasionally, for about 20 minutes or until cooked through.

4.   Taste and adjust the seasonings. Serve garnished with the slices of the fresh avocado. Bon appétit!

Nutrition Info: Per Serving: Calories: 369; Fat: 18.1g;

Carbs: 43.5g; Protein: 13.2g

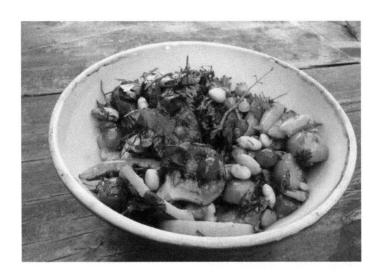

Dinner Rice & Lentils

Servings: 4

Cooking Time: 25 Minutes

Ingredients:

- 2 tbsp olive oil
- 4 scallions, chopped
- 1 carrot, diced
- 1 celery stalk, chopped
- 2 (15-oz) cans lentils, drained
- 1 (15-oz) can diced tomatoes
- 1 tbsp dried rosemary
- 1 tsp ground coriander
- 1 tbsp garlic powder
- 2 cups cooked brown rice
- Sea salt and black pepper to taste

Directions:

1. Heat the oil in a pot over medium heat. Place in scallions, carrot and celery, cook for 5 minutes until tender. Stir in lentils, tomatoes, rosemary, coriander, and garlic powder. Lower the heat and simmer for 5-7 minutes. Mix in rice, salt, and pepper and cook another 2-3 minutes. Serve.

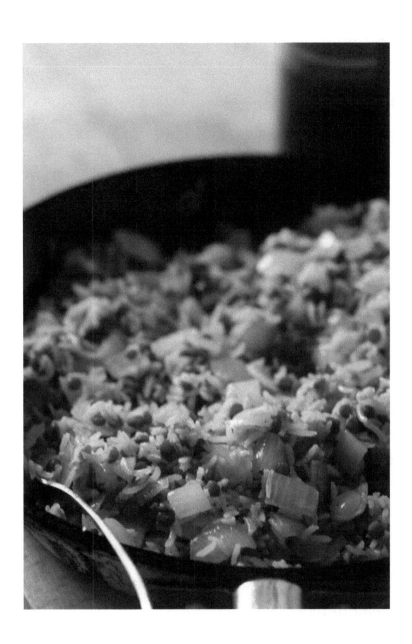

Mediterranean Tomato Gravy

Servings: 6

Cooking Time: 20 Minutes

Ingredients:

- 3 tablespoons olive oil
- 1 red onion, chopped
- 3 cloves garlic, crushed
- 4 tablespoons cornstarch
- 1 can (14 ½-ounce tomatoes, crushed
- 1/2 teaspoon dried basil
- 1/2 teaspoon dried oregano
- 1/2 teaspoon dried thyme
- 1 teaspoon dried parsley flakes
- Sea salt and black pepper, to taste

Directions:

1. Heat the olive oil in a large saucepan over medium-high heat. Once hot, sauté the onion and garlic until tender and fragrant.
2. Add in the cornstarch and continue to cook for 1 minute more.

3.	Add in the canned tomatoes and bring to a boil over medium-high heat; stir in the spices and turn the heat to a simmer.

4.	Let it simmer for about 10 minutes until everything is cooked through.

5.	Serve with vegetables of choice. Bon appétit!

Nutrition Info: Per Serving: Calories: 106; Fat: 6.6g; Carbs: 9.6g; Protein: 0.8g

Cherry & Pistachio Bulgur

Servings: 4

Cooking Time: 45 Minutes

Ingredients:

- 1 tbsp plant butter
- 1 white onion, chopped
- 1 carrot, chopped
- 1 celery stalk, chopped
- 1 cup chopped mushrooms
- 1 ½ cups bulgur
- 4 cups vegetable broth
- 1 cup chopped dried cherries, soaked
- ½ cup chopped pistachios

Directions:

1. Preheat oven to 375 F.
2. Melt butter in a skillet over medium heat. Sauté the onion, carrot and celery for 5 minutes until tender. Add in mushrooms and cook for 3 more minutes. Pour in bulgur and broth. Transfer to a casserole and bake covered for 30 minutes. Once ready, uncovered and stir in cherries. Top with pistachios to serve.

Cheesy Cauliflower Casserole

Servings: 4

Cooking Time: 35 Minutes

Ingredients:

- 2 oz plant butter
- 1 white onion, finely chopped
- ½ cup celery stalks, finely chopped
- 1 green bell pepper, chopped
- Salt and black pepper to taste
- 1 small head cauliflower, chopped
- 1 cup tofu mayonnaise
- 4 oz grated plant-based Parmesan
- 1 tsp red chili flakes

Directions:

1. Preheat oven to 400 F. Season onion, celery, and bell pepper with salt and black pepper. In a bowl, mix cauliflower, tofu mayonnaise, Parmesan cheese, and red chili flakes. Pour the mixture into a greased baking dish and add the vegetables; mix to distribute. Bake for 20 minutes. Remove and serve warm.

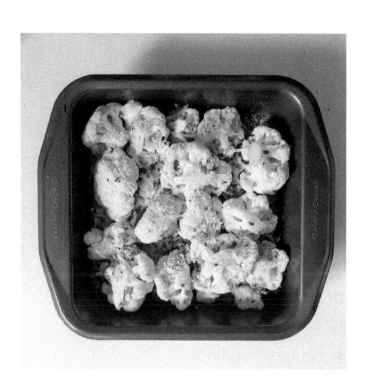

Grilled Seitan with Creole Sauce

Servings: 4

Cooking Time: 14 Minutes

Ingredients:

* Grilled Seitan Kebabs:
* 4 cups seitan, diced
* 2 medium onions, diced into squares
* 8 bamboo skewers
* 1 can coconut milk
* 2½ tablespoons creole spice
* 2 tablespoons tomato paste
* 2 cloves of garlic
* Creole Spice Mix:
* 2 tablespoons paprika
* 12 dried peri peri chili peppers
* 1 tablespoon salt
* 1 tablespoon freshly ground pepper
* 2 teaspoons dried thyme
* 2 teaspoons dried oregano

Directions:

1. Prepare the creole seasoning by blending all its ingredients and preserve in a sealable jar.

2. Thread seitan and onion on the bamboo skewers in an alternating pattern.

3. On a baking sheet, mix coconut milk with creole seasoning, tomato paste and garlic.

4. Soak the skewers in the milk marinade for 2 hours.

5. Prepare and set up a grill over medium heat.

6. Grill the skewers for 7 minutes per side.

7. Serve.

Mediterranean-style Rice

Servings: 4

Cooking Time: 20 Minutes

Ingredients:

- 3 tablespoons vegan butter, at room temperature
- 4 tablespoons scallions, chopped
- 2 cloves garlic, minced
- 1 bay leaf
- 1 thyme sprig, chopped
- 1 rosemary sprig, chopped
- 1 ½ cups white rice
- 2 cups vegetable broth
- 1 large tomato, pureed
- Sea salt and ground black pepper, to taste
- 2 ounces Kalamata olives, pitted and sliced

Directions:

1. In a saucepan, melt the vegan butter over a moderately high flame. Cook the scallions for about 2 minutes or until tender.

2. Add in the garlic, bay leaf, thyme and rosemary and continue to sauté for about 1 minute or until aromatic.

3.   Add in the rice, broth and pureed tomato. Bring to a boil; immediately turn the heat to a gentle simmer.

4.   Cook for about 15 minutes or until all the liquid has absorbed. Fluff the rice with a fork, season with salt and pepper and garnish with olives; serve immediately.

5.   Bon appétit!

Nutrition Info: Per Serving: Calories: 403; Fat: 12g; Carbs: 64.1g; Protein: 8.3g

Teff Salad with Avocado and Beans

Servings: 2

Cooking Time: 20 Minutes

Ingredients:

- 2 cups water
- 1/2 cup teff grain
- 1 teaspoon fresh lemon juice
- 3 tablespoons vegan mayonnaise
- 1 teaspoon deli mustard
- 1 small avocado, pitted, peeled and sliced
- 1 small red onion, thinly sliced
- 1 small Persian cucumber, sliced
- 1/2 cup canned kidney beans, drained
- 2 cups baby spinach

Directions:

1. In a deep saucepan, bring the water to a boil over high heat. Add in the teff grain and turn the heat to a simmer.

2. Continue to cook, covered, for about minutes or until tender. Let it cool completely.

3. Add in the remaining ingredients and toss to combine. Serve at room temperature. Bon appétit!

Nutrition Info: Per Serving: Calories: 463; Fat: 21.2g;

Carbs: 58.9g; Protein: 13.1g

Chocolate And Cherry Smoothie

Servings: 2

Cooking Time: 0 Minute

Ingredients:

- 4 cups frozen cherries
- 2 tablespoons cocoa powder
- 1 scoop of protein powder
- 1 teaspoon maple syrup
- 2 cups almond milk, unsweetened

Directions:

1. Place all the ingredients in the order in a food processor or blender and then pulse for 2 to 3 minutes at high speed until smooth.

2. Pour the smoothie into two glasses and then serve.

Nutrition Info: Calories: 324 Cal; Fat: 5 g, Carbs: 75.1 g; Protein: 7.2 g; Fiber: 11.3 g

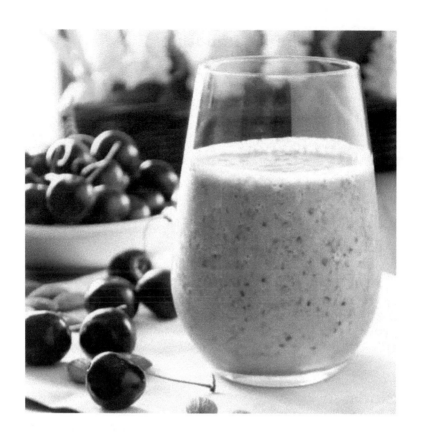

Overnight Oatmeal with Walnuts

Servings: 3

Cooking Time: 5 Minutes

Ingredients:

- 1 cup old-fashioned oats
- 3 tablespoons chia seeds • 1 ½ cups coconut milk
- 3 teaspoons agave syrup
- 1 teaspoon vanilla extract
- 1/2 teaspoon ground cinnamon
- 3 tablespoons walnuts, chopped
- A pinch of salt
- A pinch of grated nutmeg

Directions:

1. Divide the ingredients between three mason jars.
2. Cover and shake to combine well. Let them sit overnight in your refrigerator.
3. You can add some extra milk before serving.

Enjoy!

Nutrition Info: Per Serving: Calories: 423; Fat: 16.8g;

Carbs: 53.1g; Protein: 17.3g

Sesame Roasted Broccoli with Brown Rice

Servings: 4

Cooking Time: 30 Minutes

Ingredients:

- 1 head broccoli, cut into florets
- 2 tbsp olive oil
- ¾ cup pure date sugar
- ⅔ cup water
- ⅓ cup apple cider vinegar
- 1 tbsp ketchup
- ¼ cup soy sauce
- 2 tbsp cornstarch
- 4 cups cooked brown rice
- 2 scallions, chopped
- Sesame seeds

Directions:

1.   Preheat oven to 420 F. Line with parchment paper a baking sheet. Coat the broccoli with oil in a bowl. Spread on the baking sheet and roast for 20 minutes, turning once.

2.   Add the sugar, water, vinegar, and ketchup in a skillet and bring to a boil. Lower the heat and simmer for

5 minutes. In a bowl, whisk the soy sauce with cornstarch and pour into the skillet. Stir for 4 minutes. Once the broccoli is ready, transfer into the skillet and toss to combine. Share the rice into 4 bowls and top with the broccoli. Serve garnished with scallions and sesame seeds.

Tofu Eggplant Pizza

Servings: 4

Cooking Time: 45 Minutes

Ingredients:

- 2 eggplants, sliced lengthwise
- 1/3 cup melted plant butter
- 2 garlic cloves, minced
- 1 red onion
- 12 oz crumbled tofu
- 7 oz tomato sauce
- ½ tsp cinnamon powder
- 1 cup grated plant-based Parmesan
- ¼ cup chopped fresh oregano

Directions:

1.   Preheat oven to 400 F and line a baking sheet with parchment paper. Brush eggplants with some plant butter. Transfer to the baking sheet and bake until lightly browned, about 20 minutes.

2.   Heat the remaining butter in a skillet and sauté the garlic and onion until fragrant and soft, about 3 minutes. Stir in the tofu and cook for 3 minutes. Add the tomato sauce and season with salt and black pepper.

Simmer for 10 minutes.

3.   Remove the eggplant from the oven and spread the tofu sauce on top. Sprinkle with the plant-based Parmesan cheese and oregano. Bake further for 10 minutes or until the cheese has melted. Serve.

Citrus Asparagus

Servings: 4

Cooking Time: 15 Minutes

Ingredients:

- 1 onion, minced
- 2 tsp lemon zest
- 1/3 cup fresh lemon juice
- 1 tbsp olive oil
- Salt and black pepper to taste
- 1 pound asparagus, trimmed

Directions:

1. Combine the onion, lemon zest, lemon juice, and oil in a bowl. Sprinkle with salt and pepper. Let sit for 5-minutes.

2. Insert a steamer basket and 1 cup of water in a pot over medium heat. Place the asparagus on the basket and steam for 4-5 minutes until tender but crispy. Leave to cool for 10 minutes, then arrange on a plate. Serve drizzled with the dressing.

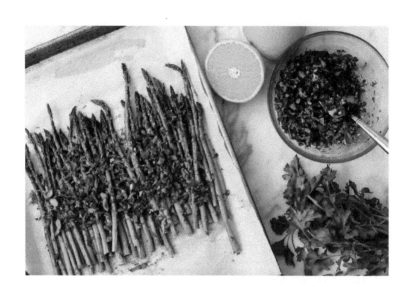

Pistachio Dip

Servings: 8

Cooking Time: 0 Minute

Ingredients:

* 2 tbsp. lemon juice • 1 t. extra virgin olive oil
* 2 tbsp. of the following:
* tahini
* parsley, chopped
* 2 cloves of garlic
* ½ c. pistachios shelled
* 15 oz. garbanzo beans, save the liquid from the can
* Salt and pepper to taste

Directions:

1. Using a food processor, add pistachios, pepper, sea salt, lemon juice, olive oil, tahini, parsley, garlic, and garbanzo beans. Pulse until mixed.

2. Using the liquid from the garbanzo beans, add to the dip while slowly blending until it reaches your desired consistency.

3. Enjoy at room temperature or warmed.

Salsa

Servings: 1 To 1 ½ Cups Cooking

Time: 5 Minutes

Ingredients:

- Pinch of salt
- Pinch of black, ground pepper
- 1 tablespoon of extra-virgin olive oil
- ½ tablespoon of lime juice
- 1 clove of garlic, diced
- 1 shallot, diced
- 1 cup of cherry tomatoes
- 1 jalapeno pepper, seeds removed and diced
- ¼ cup of cilantro

Directions:

1. Add all ingredients into a blender, pulse until coarsely chopped or smooth depending on your preference. Serve while fresh!

2. Tips:

3. Add bell peppers or pineapple for a twist to this delicious salsa recipe.

4. For a spicier salsa, leave the jalapeno seeds intact.

Burrito-stuffed Sweet Potatoes

Servings: 4

Cooking Time: 45 Minutes

Ingredients:

- For Sweet Potatoes:
- 1 cup cooked black beans
- 4 small sweet potatoes
- ½ cup of brown rice
- ½ teaspoon minced garlic
- 1 teaspoon tomato paste
- 1 teaspoon ground cumin
- ¼ teaspoon salt
- ½ teaspoon olive oil
- 1 ¼ cup water
- For the Salsa:
- 1 cup cherry tomatoes, halved
- 1 medium red bell pepper, deseeded, chopped
- ¾ cup chopped red onion
- 2 tablespoon chopped cilantro leaves
- ½ teaspoon salt
- ¼ teaspoon ground black pepper
- 1 ½ teaspoon olive oil

- 1 tablespoon lime juice
- For the Guacamole:
- 1 medium avocado, pitted, peeled
- ½ teaspoon minced garlic
- 2 tablespoons chopped cilantro leaves
- ¼ teaspoon salt •   1 tablespoon lime juice
- For Serving:
- Shredded cabbage as needed

Directions:

1. Prepare sweet potatoes and for this, place them in a baking dish, prick them with a fork and bake for 45 minutes at 400 degrees F until very tender.

2. Meanwhile, place a medium saucepan over medium heat, add rice and beans, stir in salt, oil, and tomatoes paste, pour in water and bring the mixture to boil.

3. Switch heat to medium-low level, simmer for 40 minutes until all the liquid has absorbed and set aside until required.

4. Prepare the salsa and for this, place all its ingredients in a bowl and stir until combined, set aside until required.

5.   Prepare the guacamole and for this, place the avocado in a bowl, mash well, then add remaining ingredients, stir until combined, and set aside until required.

6.   When sweet potatoes are baked, cut them along the top, pull back the skin, then split and top with rice and beans mixture.

7.   Top with salsa and guacamole and cabbage and serve.

Nutrition Info: Calories: 388 Cal; Fat: 11 g: Carbs: 67.1 g; Protein: 10.5 g; Fiber: 15.7 g

Broccoli And White Beans with Potatoes and Walnuts

Servings: 4

Cooking Time: 35 Minutes

Ingredients:

- 1½ pounds fingerling potatoes
- 4 cups broccoli florets
- 3 tablespoons extra-virgin olive oil
- 3 garlic cloves, minced
- ¾ cup chopped walnut pieces
- ¼ teaspoon crushed red pepper
- 1½ cups or 1 (15.5-ounce) can white beans, drained and rinsed
- 1 teaspoon dried savory
- Salt and freshly ground black pepper
- 1 tablespoon fresh lemon juice

Directions:

1. Preparing the Ingredients
2. Steam the potatoes until tender for about minutes. Set aside.
3. Steam the broccoli until crisp-tender. Set aside.

4. In a large skillet, heat 2 tablespoons of the oil over medium heat. Add the garlic, walnuts, and crushed red pepper. Cook until the garlic is softened.

5. Stir in the steamed potatoes and broccoli. Add the beans and savory, then season with salt and black pepper. Cook until heated through.

6. Finish and Serve

7. Sprinkle with lemon juice and drizzle with the remaining 1 tablespoon olive oil.

8. Serve immediately.

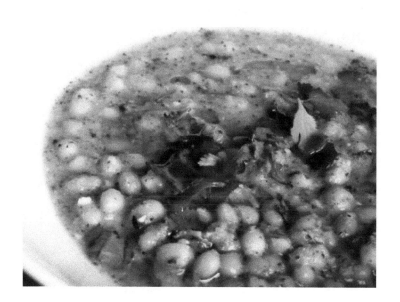

Lentil Meatballs with Coconut Curry Sauce

Servings: 14

Cooking Time: 60 Minutes

Ingredients:

- For the Lentil Meatballs:
- 6 ounces tofu, firm, drained
- 1 cup black lentils
- ½ cup quinoa
- 1 teaspoon garlic powder
- 1 teaspoon salt
- 1/3 cup chopped cilantro
- 1 teaspoon fennel seed
- 1 Tablespoon olive oil
- For the Curry:
- 1 large tomato, diced
- 2 teaspoons minced garlic
- 1 tablespoon grated ginger
- 1 teaspoon brown sugar
- ½ teaspoon ground turmeric
- ¼ teaspoon cayenne pepper
- ½ teaspoon salt
- ¼ teaspoon ground black pepper
- 1 tablespoon lime juice

- 2 tablespoons olive oil
- 1 tablespoon dried fenugreek leaves
- 13.5 ounces coconut milk, unsweetened

Directions:

1. Boil lentils and fennel in 3 cups water over high heat, then simmer for 25 minutes, and when done, drain them and set aside until required.

2. Meanwhile, boil the quinoa in 1 cup water over high heat and then simmer for 15 minutes over low heat until cooked.

3. Prepare the sauce and for this, place a pot over medium heat, add oil, ginger, and garlic, cook for 2 minutes, then stir in turmeric, cook for 1 minute, add tomatoes and cook for 5 minutes.

4. Add remaining ingredients for the sauce, stir until mixed and simmer until ready to serve.

5. Transfer half of the lentils in a food processor, add quinoa and pulse until the mixture resembles sand.

6. Tip the mixture into a bowl, add remaining ingredients for the meatballs and stir until well mixed.

7. Place tofu in a food processor, add 1 tablespoon oil, process until the smooth paste comes together, add

to lentil mixture, stir until well mixed and shape the mixture into small balls.

8.   Place the balls on a baking sheet, spray with oil and bake for 20 minutes until golden brown.

9.   Add balls into the warm sauce, toss until coated, sprinkle with cilantro, and serve.

Nutrition Info: Calories: 150.8 Cal; Fat: 4.6 g: Carbs: 18 g; Protein: 10.2 g; Fiber: 6.8 g

Anasazi Bean and Vegetable Stew

Servings: 3

Cooking Time: 1 Hour

Ingredients:

- 1 cup Anasazi beans, soaked overnight and drained
- 3 cups roasted vegetable broth
- 1 bay laurel
- 1 thyme sprig, chopped
- 1 rosemary sprig, chopped
- 3 tablespoons olive oil
- 1 large onion, chopped
- 2 celery stalks, chopped
- 2 carrots, chopped
- 2 bell peppers, seeded and chopped
- 1 green chili pepper, seeded and chopped
- 2 garlic cloves, minced
- Sea salt and ground black pepper, to taste
- 1 teaspoon cayenne pepper
- 1 teaspoon paprika

Directions:

1.   In a saucepan, bring the Anasazi beans and broth to a boil. Once boiling, turn the heat to a simmer. Add in the bay laurel, thyme and rosemary; let it cook for about 50 minutes or until tender.

2.   Meanwhile, in a heavy-bottomed pot, heat the olive oil over medium-high heat. Now, sauté the onion, celery, carrots and peppers for about 4 minutes until tender.

3.   Add in the garlic and continue to sauté for seconds more or until aromatic.

4.   Add the sautéed mixture to the cooked beans. Season with salt, black pepper, cayenne pepper and paprika.

5.   Continue to simmer, stirring periodically, for 10 minutes more or until everything is cooked through. Bon appétit!

Nutrition Info: Per Serving: Calories: 444; Fat: 15.8g;

Carbs: 58.2g; Protein: 20.2g

Mexican-style Bean Bowl

Servings: 6

Cooking Time: 1 Hour

Ingredients:

- 1 pound red beans, soaked overnight and drained
- 1 cup canned corn kernels, drained
- 2 roasted bell peppers, sliced
- 1 chili pepper, finely chopped
- 1 cup cherry tomatoes, halved
- 1 red onion, chopped
- 1/4 cup fresh cilantro, chopped
- 1/4 cup fresh parsley, chopped
- 1 teaspoon Mexican oregano
- 1/4 cup red wine vinegar
- 2 tablespoons fresh lemon juice
- 1/3 cup extra-virgin olive oil
- Sea salt and ground black, to taste
- 1 avocado, peeled, pitted and sliced

Directions:

1. Cover the soaked beans with a fresh change of cold water and bring to a boil. Let it boil for about

minutes. Turn the heat to a simmer and continue to cook for 50 to 55 minutes or until tender.

2. Allow your beans to cool completely, then, transfer them to a salad bowl.

3. Add in the remaining ingredients and toss to combine well. Serve at room temperature.

4. Bon appétit!

Nutrition Info: Per Serving: Calories: 465; Fat: 17.9g;

Carbs: 60.4g; Protein: 20.2g

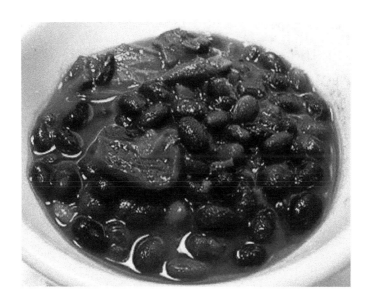

Cherry Tomato Dressing

Servings: 1

Cooking Time: 5 Minutes

Ingredients:

- ¼ teaspoon of black pepper
- ¼ teaspoon of salt
- ¼ teaspoon of garlic powder
- ½ teaspoon of onion powder
- ½ a teaspoon of paprika
- 1 tablespoon of agave nectar
- ¼ cup of olive oil
- ¼ cup of balsamic vinegar
- Cherry tomatoes

Directions:

1. Combine all the ingredients in a food processor and blend until smooth.

Old-fashioned Pecan Spread

Servings: 16

Cooking Time: 10 Minutes

Ingredients:

- 2 cups pecan, soaked and drained
- 5 tablespoons coconut oil
- 4 tablespoons orange juice
- 1 cup dates, pitted

Directions:

1. In your food processor or a high-speed blender, pulse the pecans until ground.
2. Then, process the nuts for minutes more, scraping down the sides and bottom of the bowl.
3. Add in the coconut oil, orange juice and dates. Continue to blend until your desired consistency is achieved.
4. Bon appétit!

Nutrition Info: Per Serving: Calories: 125; Fat: 13.1g;

Carbs: 2.5g; Protein: 1.1g

Spicy Steamed Broccoli

Servings: 6

Cooking Time: 15 Minutes

Ingredients:

- 1 large head broccoli, into florets
- Salt to taste
- 1 tsp red pepper flakes

Directions:

1. Boil cup water in a pot over medium heat. Place in a steamer basket and put in the florets. Steam covered for 5-7 minutes. In a bowl, toss the broccoli with red pepper flakes and salt. Serve.

Lemony Arugula with Pine Nuts

Servings: 4

Cooking Time: 20 Minutes

Ingredients:

- 2 bunches arugula, chopped
- 3 tbsp olive oil
- 3 garlic cloves, minced
- 1 tsp cayenne pepper
- Zest of 1 lemon
- ¼ cup toasted pine nuts for garnish

Directions:

1. Steam the arugula in a pot over medium heat for 2-3 minutes. Drain and set aside.

2. Heat the oil in a skillet over medium heat. Add in garlic and cook for 30 seconds. Mix in arugula, cayenne pepper, lemon zest, salt, pepper. Serve garnished with toasted pine nuts.

Sherry Shallot Beans

Servings: 5

Cooking Time: 25 Minutes

Ingredients:

- 1 tsp olive oil
- 4 shallots, chopped
- 1 tsp ground cumin
- 1 (14.5-oz) cans black beans
- 1 cup vegetable broth
- 2 tbsp sherry vinegar

Directions:

1. Heat the oil in a pot over medium heat. Place in shallots and cumin and cook for 3 minutes until soft. Stir in beans and broth. Bring to a boil, then lower the heat and simmer for minutes. Add in sherry vinegar, increase the heat and cook for an additional 3 minutes. Serve warm.

Chocolate Smoothie

Servings: 2

Cooking Time: 5 Minutes

Ingredients:

- ¼ c. almond butter
- ¼ c. cocoa powder, unsweetened
- ½ c. coconut milk, canned
- 1 c. almond milk, unsweetened

Directions:

1. Before making the smoothie, freeze the almond milk into cubes using an ice cube tray. This would take a few hours, so prepare it ahead.
2. Blend everything using your preferred machine until it reaches your desired thickness.
3. Serve immediately and enjoy!

Nutrition Info: Calories: 147 Carbohydrates: 8.2 g Proteins: 4 g Fats: 13.4 g

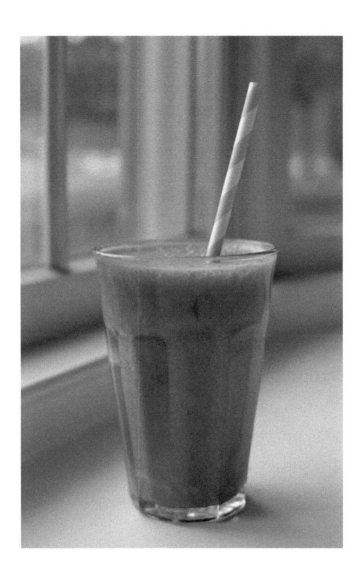

Easy Barley Risotto

Servings: 4

Cooking Time: 35 Minutes

Ingredients:

- 2 tablespoons vegan butter
- 1 medium onion, chopped
- 1 bell pepper, seeded and chopped
- 2 garlic cloves, minced
- 1 teaspoon ginger, minced
- 2 cups vegetable broth
- 2 cups water
- 1 cup medium pearl barley
- 1/2 cup white wine
- 2 tablespoons fresh chives, chopped

Directions:

1.   Melt the vegan butter in a saucepan over mediumhigh heat.

2.   Once hot, cook the onion and pepper for about 3 minutes until just tender.

3.   Add in the garlic and ginger and continue to sauté for 2 minutes or until aromatic.

4.   Add in the vegetable broth, water, barley and wine; cover and continue to simmer for about 30 minutes. Once all the liquid has been absorbed; fluff the barley with a fork.

5.   Garnish with fresh chives and serve warm. Bon appétit!

Nutrition Info: Per Serving: Calories: 269; Fat: 7.1g; Carbs: 43.9g; Protein: 8g

Vegan Ricotta Cheese

Servings: 12

Cooking Time: 10 Minutes

Ingredients:

- 1/2 cup raw cashew nuts, soaked overnight and drained
- 1/2 cup raw sunflower seeds, soaked overnight and drained
- 1/4 cup water
- 1 heaping tablespoon coconut oil, melted
- 1 tablespoon lime juice, freshly squeezed
- 1 tablespoon white vinegar
- 1/4 teaspoon Dijon mustard
- 2 tablespoons nutritional yeast
- 1/2 teaspoon garlic powder
- 1/2 teaspoon turmeric powder
- 1/2 teaspoon salt

Directions:

1. Process the cashews, sunflower seeds and water in your blender until creamy and uniform.

2. Add in the remaining ingredients; continue to blend until everything is well incorporated.

3.   Keep in your refrigerator for up to a week. Bon appétit!

Nutrition Info: Per Serving: Calories: 74; Fat: 6.3g; Carbs: 3.3g; Protein: 2.7g